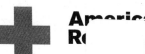

AUTOMATED EXTERNAL DEFIBRILLATION

Important certification information

American Red Cross certificates may be issued upon successful completion of a training program that uses this textbook as an integral part of the course. By itself, the text material does not constitute comprehensive Red Cross training. In order to issue ARC certificates, your instructor must be authorized by the American Red Cross and must follow prescribed policies and procedures. Make certain that you have attended a course authorized by the American Red Cross. Ask your instructor about receiving American Red Cross certification, or contact your local chapter for more information.

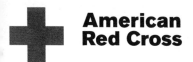

American
Red Cross

AUTOMATED EXTERNAL DEFIBRILLATION

StayWell

StayWell

**A Times Mirror
Company**

Printed in the United States of America
Composition by Progressive Information Technologies
Printing/Binding by Western Graphic Communications

StayWell
263 Summer St.
Boston, MA. 02210

Library of Congress Cataloging-in-Publication Data

Automated external defibrillation/American Red Cross.
      p.   cm.
   "This manual is based on Appendix A of the: American Red Cross emergency response, revised ed."
   ISBN 0-323-00439-3
   1. Defibrillators.   2. Electric countershock.   3. Cardiovascular emergencies—Treatment.   4. Emergency medical technicians.
I. American Red Cross.   II. American Red Cross emergency response. Rev. ed.
RC684.E4A95 1998
616.1'23025—dc21   98–14957
                                            CIP

98 99 00 01 02 / 9 8 7 6 5 4 3 2

Acknowledgments

his manual is based on Appendix A of the *American Red Cross Emergency Response Revised Edition* (Stock No. 656501). We developed this course through the careful consideration of the latest research information, technology, comments of reviewers, and feedback from those who teach automated external defibrillation or those who work in an out-of-hospital environment. Without the commitment to excellence from both paid and volunteer staff, this manual could not have been created.

Members of the Automated External Defibrillation project development team responsible for designing this course and writing this manual included the following: Jose V. Salazar, MPH, NREMT-P, Project Team Leader; Rhonda Starr, Project Manager; Mike Espino, Don K. Vardell, MS, Senior Associates; Thomas Bates, NREMT-B, Jon Patrick Ewing, Gary Horewitz, JD, NREMT-P, Steve Lynch, and Jane Moore, Associates, New Products and Services Development; Don May, Senior Associate, Greg Stockton, Associate, Product and Services Support; Earl Harbert, Manager, Contract and Financial Management; CP Dail, Jr., Senior Associate; Amy Janocha, Associate, Business Planning and Development; Marietta Damond, Senior Associate, Program Evaluation. Administrative Support was provided by Betty Butler and Vivian Mills.

The following American Red Cross national headquarters Chapter Operations staff provided guidance and review: Mark Robinson, Vice President, Anthony Gallagher, Manager, Program Evaluation; Dana Jessen, Manager, Product and Services Support.

The Mosby Editorial and Production Team included: Claire Merrick, Editor-in-Chief; Christine Ambrose, Managing Editor; Shannon Bates and Nadine Steffan, Project Supervisors; Jerry Wood, Director of Manufacturing; Betty Mueller, Manufacturing Manager; Theresa Fuchs, Manager, Media Relations.

Guidance and review were also provided by members of the AED Project Ad Hoc group:

Suzanne P. Hulette
Director of Educational Services
Central Georgia Chapter
Macon, GA

Richard Myers, NREMT-P
Alexandria Fire Department
Sterling, VA

Paul Roman
Chairman, ASTM, F30.02.03 Task Group on First
    Responders
Executive Director
New Jersey EMT Registry
American Red Cross
Board Member
Jersey Coast Chapter
Shrewsbury, NJ

Alonzo W. Smith, BA, NREMT-P
National Council of State EMS Training Coordinators, Inc.
Columbia, SC

John Van Rieg
Assistant Director of Health and Safety for Workplace
    Programs
Greater Houston Area Chapter
Houston, TX

Dr. Peter Wernicki
United States Life Saving Association
Vero Beach, FL

Additional external review was provided by—

Mark Altman
Manager of Customer Education
SurVivaLink Corp.
Minnetonka, MN

Craig Aman
Training Development Manager
Heartstream
Seattle, WA

Linda Del Monte
Clinical Manager
Physio-Control Corporation
Redmond, WA

Chris D'Esposito
Marketing Specialist
Laerdal Medical Corporation
Wappingers Falls, NY

John Nealon
Director of Marketing
SurVivaLink Corporation
Minnetonka, MN

Al Weigel
Director of Marketing
Laerdal Medical Corporation
Wappingers Falls, NY

**Special thanks go to Rick Brady, Photographer
and the Town of Leesburg Police Department
Leesburg, Virginia.**

How to Use This Manual

The Automated External Defibrillation manual—

- Is an integral part of the American Red Cross Automated External Defibrillation (AED) Training course designed to help you learn how to properly and safely use an AED for victims in cardiac arrest.
- Is designed to help you learn and understand the material it presents. It includes the following features:
  - Objectives that describe what you should know and be able to do after reading the manual and participating in class activities. Read these objectives carefully and refer back to them from time to time as you read the manual.
  - A full-color skill sheet describes how to perform the skill that you need to be able to demonstrate at the completion of this course.
  - A glossary, providing definitions to terms in the manual that may be unfamiliar. All glossary terms appear in the manual in bold type the first time they are used or explained.
- Is designed for individuals trained in professional rescuer-level CPR. Contact your local Red Cross for course information.

Contents

Objectives

fter reading this material, you should be able to—

- Describe the rationale for early defibrillation.
- Describe the abnormal heart rhythms commonly present during cardiac arrest.
- Explain what defibrillation is and how it works.
- Discuss when defibrillation is appropriate and when it is not.
- Explain the role of CPR in cardiac arrest.
- Explain the general differences between manual and automated external defibrillation.
- Identify the general steps for the use of an automated external defibrillator (AED).
- List precautions for the use of an AED.
- Identify special resuscitation situations that can arise when using an AED.
- Identify elements that should be considered when establishing an early defibrillation program.

After reading this material and completing the appropriate course activities, you should be able to—

- Demonstrate how to properly use an AED in a cardiac arrest situation.
- Demonstrate the ability to make appropriate decisions while using an AED for a victim of cardiac arrest.

Introduction

Each year, approximately 500,000 adult Americans die as a result of coronary disease. Almost half of these deaths occur suddenly, from cardiac arrest. Most of these arrests occur away from a hospital, where the care needed to immediately correct the cardiac arrest condition is not readily available. CPR, started promptly, can help by keeping oxygen flowing to the brain. However, in many cases CPR by itself is insufficient to correct the underlying heart problem. What is needed to correct the problem, in many sudden cardiac arrests, is an electric shock. The sooner the shock is administered, the greater the likelihood of the victim's survival.

In the out-of-hospital setting, this shock, known as **defibrillation,** has typically been administered only by paramedics. But paramedics are rarely the first to arrive on the emergency scene. Often, EMT-Basics and first responders, such as fire fighters, law enforcement personnel, and lifeguards, arrive first or are already on the scene. But without the capability to defibrillate victims of cardiac arrest, they are limited to performing CPR while awaiting the arrival of more advanced personnel. This delay in defibrillation is believed to be a major contributing factor to the low survival rate associated with out-of-hospital cardiac arrest.

As a result of this low survival rate, the medical community is refocusing efforts on providing earlier defibrillation to cardiac arrest victims. To make earlier defibrillation possible, both the defibrillator and the skills needed to properly operate it have been simplified. Simplification has resulted in more individuals being able to defibrillate cardiac arrest victims and more victims of cardiac arrest being saved. This program has been developed to help train responders about the basic principles of how automated external defibrillators work, how to use them, and why defibrillation programs are needed.

The Heart's Electrical System

To better understand both the limitations of CPR and how defibrillation works, it is helpful to understand how the heart's electrical system functions. The electrical system determines the pumping action of the heart. Under normal conditions, specialized cells of the heart initiate and carry on electrical activity. These cells make up what is commonly called the **conduction system.** Think of the conduction system as the pathway or road that electrical impulses must travel. This pathway originates in the upper chambers of the heart, known as the **atria.** It ends in the lower chambers of the heart, known as the **ventricles** (Fig. 1).

The normal point of origin of the electrical impulse is the **sinoatrial (SA) node.** Approximately every second of an adult's life, a new electrical impulse is generated from the SA node. This impulse travels down the pathway of cells to a point midway between the atria and ventricles. This point is the **atrioventricular (AV) node.**

Below the AV node the pathway divides, like a fork in a road, into two branches. The electrical im-

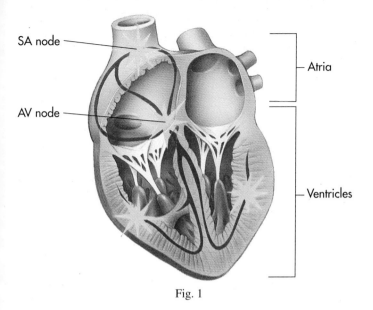

Fig. 1

pulse travels by way of these right and left bundle branches to its final destination, the right and left ventricles.

These right and left bundle branches become a vast network of microscopic fibers, called **Purkinje fibers,** which spread electrical impulses across the heart. Under normal conditions, this impulse reaches the muscular walls of the ventricles and causes the ventricles to contract. The strong contraction of the ventricles forces blood out of the heart to circulate through the body. The contraction of the left ventricle results in a pulse. The pauses between the pulse beats you feel are the periods between contractions.

Through the timing of these electrical impulses, the chambers of the heart are able to contract and relax. When they contract, blood is forced out of the heart. When they relax, blood refills the chambers.

The electrical activity of the heart can be evaluated by a cardiac monitor or **electrocardiograph.** A cardiac monitor has electrodes that usually are attached to the chest. The electrodes pick up the electrical impulse and transmit it to the monitor. The movement of the electrical impulse down the pathway appears as a graphic record on the monitor. This graphic record is referred to as an **electrocardiogram (ECG).** A regular rhythm that occurs within a normal rate, 60 to 100 beats per minute (bpm), and without unusual variations, is called a **normal sinus rhythm.** This rhythm appears on an ECG as a series of regularly spaced and sized peaks and valleys (Fig. 2A).

When the Heart Fails

Any damage to the heart, caused either by disease or injury, can disrupt the conduction system. This disruption can result in an abnormal heart rhythm that can stop circulation. The two most common abnormal rhythms that are present initially in cardiac arrest victims are ventricular tachycardia (V-tach) and ventricular fibrillation (V-fib). **Ventricular fibrillation** is a state of totally disorganized electrical activity in the heart (Fig. 2B). It results in the fibrillation, or quivering, of the ven-

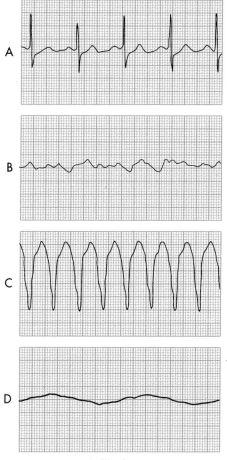

Fig. 2

tricles. This fibrillation is not adequate for the ventricles to pump blood. Consequently, there is no pulse.

Ventricular tachycardia refers to a very rapid contraction of the ventricles. Though there is electrical activity resulting in a regular rhythm, the rate is often so fast that the heart is unable to pump blood properly (Fig. 2C). As with V-fib, when blood flow is severely impaired, there will not be a pulse.

Defibrillation

In many cases, these two abnormal rhythms can be corrected by early defibrillation. During defibrillation, an electrical shock is delivered to the heart. This shock is intended to disrupt abnormal electrical activity, such as that of V-fib and V-tach, long enough to allow the heart to spontaneously develop an effective rhythm on its own.

If not interrupted, these rhythms will deteriorate to the point where all electrical activity will cease, a condition known as **asystole** (Fig. 2D). Asystole is not corrected by defibrillation. However, CPR is still important for a heart in asystole. Remember, you will not be able to tell what, if any, rhythm the heart is in by feeling for a pulse.

The role of CPR

CPR, begun immediately and continued until defibrillation is available, helps maintain a low level of circulation in the body until the abnormal rhythms are corrected by defibrillation. In addition, CPR performed during this period maintains vital organs, such as the brain. However, CPR cannot maintain this low-level circulation indefinitely and cannot convert V-fib or V-tach to a normal sinus rhythm. The major factor determining survival for a person in V-fib is the time until defibrillation. The longer the wait, the poorer the outcome. For this reason, programs teaching and promoting early CPR and defibrillation to more emergency care providers, such as first responders, are encouraged.

Automated External Defibrillators: Improving Survival of Cardiac Arrest

The use of the traditional manual defibrillator requires specialized training that includes learning how to recognize abnormal rhythms on a monitor and how to deliver a shock with hand-held paddles. The process demands extensive training, and manual defibrillators are expensive. It is impractical to train first responders in their use.

Instead, the answer to the problem of how to get timely, lifesaving defibrillation to cardiac arrest victims as soon as possible lies with **automated external defibrillators (AEDs)** (Fig. 3). As the name implies, the AED is an automated device capable of automatically recognizing a heart rhythm that requires a shock. It can then charge itself and prompt the rescuer to deliver a shock to the victim by pressing a button. These devices are sometimes referred to as SAEDs.

AEDs are simple to operate and extremely reliable when used properly. AEDs analyze the victim's

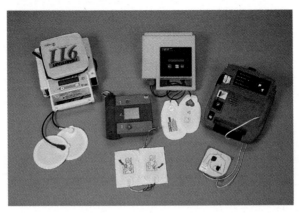

Fig. 3

heart rhythm several times before identifying it as a shockable rhythm.

Using an automated external defibrillator (AED)

In a situation involving cardiac arrest, an AED should be put to use as soon as it is available and safe to do so. CPR in progress must be stopped once the AED is applied. All AEDs can be operated by following five simple steps:

1. Confirm cardiac arrest. Check for unresponsiveness and the absence of breathing and pulse.
2. Attach the AED to defibrillator pads and cables and turn on the AED. Apply the pads to the victim's bare chest.
3. Let the AED analyze the heart rhythm (or push the button marked "analyze").
4. Advise all rescuers & bystanders to "stand clear."
5. Deliver a shock by pushing the shock button if indicated and prompted by the AED.

42351

Whether you are the first person to arrive on the scene or arrive after CPR has been started, you should check the victim's pulse to determine that the victim is actually in cardiac arrest before attaching the AED (Fig. 4). The absence of a pulse confirms cardiac arrest. When you establish the absence of a pulse, you should turn on the AED (Fig. 5). Once turned on, some AEDs are capable of recording the events surrounding the care of the victim. If the AED you are using has a voice recording mechanism, you should briefly give a verbal report for the recording. It should include —

- Your identity and location.
- Assessment findings.
- Any significant events that have occurred (such as a drowning incident or trauma).

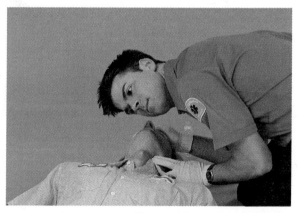

Fig. 4

Next, prepare to attach the electrode pads to the victim's chest. To do this, the victim's chest must be bare and wiped dry.

- Remove the pads from their packaging.
- If needed, connect the two cables from the AED to the pads (Fig. 6). Peel away the protective plastic backing from the pads (Fig. 7).
- Wipe the victim's chest dry, if needed.
- Place the pads, adhesive-side down, on the victim's chest.
- Place one pad on the upper-right side of the victim's chest, above the nipple and below the collarbone.
- Place the other pad on the lower-left side of the victim's chest, below the nipple (Fig. 8).

If you are confused about which pad goes where, remember the phrase "white on right." This means that the pad attached to the white cable is

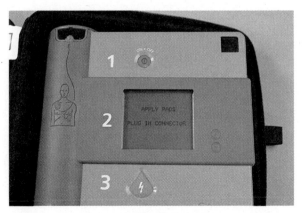

Fig. 5

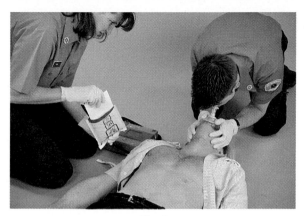

Fig. 6

applied to the upper-right side of the victim's chest. However, some AEDs may not have color-coded cables, in which case either pad can go in either location on the chest.

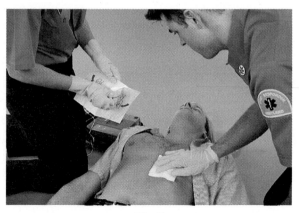

Fig. 7

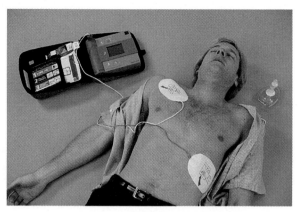

Fig. 8

If the pads are not securely attached to the chest or if the cables are not fastened properly, you will receive a connect electrodes message from the AED. This message may appear in print on the small screen on the front of the machine and/or in voice prompt. If you receive such a message, check to see that the pads and cables are attached properly. In all cases, you must follow the manufacturer's instructions, since AEDs differ in the type of cables and adhesive pads used.

At this point, the AED is ready to analyze the heart rhythm. Some devices require the first responder to press the button marked "analyze" to have the machine examine the heart rhythm. Other models will automatically analyze the heart rhythm (Fig. 9). Be sure no one is touching or moving the victim during this time. If the AED identifies a rhythm that should be defibrillated, it will prompt you with either an on-screen message or by voice prompt, or

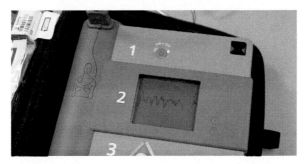

Fig. 9

both. This message often states "shock advised," followed by "press to shock," indicating that you need to press a button to defibrillate the victim (Fig. 10).

You will also be instructed by a voice prompt from the AED to "stand clear" before administering a shock. This is an important measure that you and others present must follow. Anytime an AED is

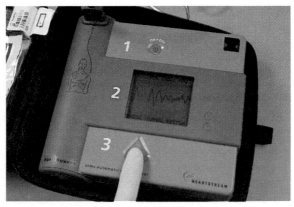

Fig. 10

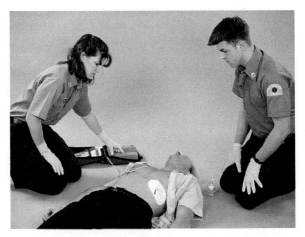

Fig. 11

analyzing the rhythm, charging to a specific energy level, or delivering a shock, *you and others must not be in contact with the victim* (Fig. 11). It is the responsibility of the operator to warn and move rescuers away from contact with the victim before analyzing and before depressing the shock button. This can be done by shouting "stand clear." Another common warning is "I'm clear, you're clear, everybody clear" while actually checking around the victim before pressing the shock button.

The number of shocks the AED administers and the energy level for each shock is often preset by the manufacturer according to standard of care set by the local medical director. The local medical director can establish local operating protocols. The American Heart Association has established guidelines to follow when using an AED. These guidelines include how CPR is to be used as part of the protocol.

Sample AED Protocol

Check Pulse

If no pulse . . . Do CPR until AED is attached.

Analyze Rhythm

If shock advised . . . Defibrillate.

Analyze Rhythm

If shock advised . . . Defibrillate.

Analyze Rhythm

If shock advised . . . Defibrillate.

Recheck Pulse

If no pulse . . . Do 1 minute of CPR and recheck pulse.

If still no pulse . . . Repeat analysis and set of 3 shocks.

Recheck Pulse

If no pulse . . . Do 1 minute of CPR and recheck pulse.

If still no pulse . . . Repeat analysis and set of 3 shocks
as indicated.

Recheck Pulse

If still no pulse . . . Continue CPR and prepare to transport.

Note: As long as the pulse is absent and the AED still indicates a need to shock, continue repeating sets of 3 shocks to the maximum your local protocol allows, with 1 minute of CPR between each set. You should be thoroughly familiar with your local operating procedures, which may vary slightly from this table.

In some instances, the heart will *not* require defibrillation. In this case, the device will inform you that no shock is needed and you should recheck the victim's pulse. Leave the AED attached to the victim. If the pulse is still absent, resume CPR. If a pulse is present, recheck breathing. If the victim is still not breathing, continue breathing for the victim and monitoring the pulse.

Precautions

You need to take the following precautions when using an AED:

- Do not use alcohol pads to clean the chest before attaching the pads. The alcohol is flammable.
- Stand clear of the victim while analyzing and defibrillating.
- Do not analyze the rhythm or defibrillate in a moving vehicle.
- Do not defibrillate a victim who is in water. Move victims away from puddles of water (such as around a swimming pool) before defibrillating.
- Do not defibrillate a victim lying on a surface, such as sheet metal, that is likely to transfer the electrical energy to others on or in contact with the same surface.
- Do not defibrillate a victim who is less than 8 years old or weighs less than 90 pounds (follow your local protocols).
- Do not defibrillate a victim while he or she is wearing a medication patch on the chest. Remove any patch from the chest with a gloved hand, and wipe the area clean before attaching the device.
- Do not defibrillate someone in the presence of flammable materials (such as gasoline).

- Avoid radio transmissions while defibrillating, including cell phones within 6 feet of the victim.
- Keep breathing devices with free flowing oxygen away from the victim during defibrillation.

Special Resuscitation Situations

Some situations require rescuers to pay special attention when using an AED. It is important that rescuers be familiar with these situations and be able to respond appropriately.

AEDs around water

When using an AED near the water, such as at a pool facility, you should attempt to put the victim on a dry surface such as a backboard. The victim's chest should be wiped dry. If possible, the victim should be placed on a backboard and moved away from the water. Proceed to use the defibrillator as in any situation.

If you are outdoors and it is raining, you should move the victim somewhere away from the rain, such as under an awning. Then wipe the chest dry.

AEDs and pacemakers

People whose hearts are weak and not able to generate an electrical impulse may have a pacemaker implanted. The pacemaker serves the function of the SA node (see p. 3). These small implantable devices may sometimes be located in the area below the right collar bone. There may be a small lump that can be felt under the skin. Sometimes the pacemaker is placed somewhere else.

If visible, or you know that the victim has a pacemaker, do not place the defibrillation pads directly over the pacemaker. This may interfere with the delivery of the shock. Adjust pad placement and continue to follow the protocol. If you are not sure, use the AED, if needed. It will not harm the victim or rescuer.

AEDs for infants and children

Cardiac arrest in infants and children mainly results from respiratory failure, not cardiac failure. Therefore, clearing the airway is the main focus of any infant or child resuscitation. AEDs on the market are not designed for infants and children. These machines do not have the capability to adjust to the low energy settings needed for infants and children. If you are dealing with an infant or child in cardiac arrest, initiate CPR and call for more advanced medical care.

Nitroglycerin patches and AEDs

People that have a history of cardiac problems may use nitroglycerin patches (Nitropatch®) (Fig. 12). These patches are usually placed on the chest. If you encounter a victim with a patch on his or her chest, remove it, preferably with a gloved hand. Nitroglycerin patches look very similar to nicotine patches that people use to stop smoking. Although these patches do not interfere with defibrillation, time may be wasted attempting to identify the type of patch. Therefore, any medication patches that are on the victim's chest should be removed.

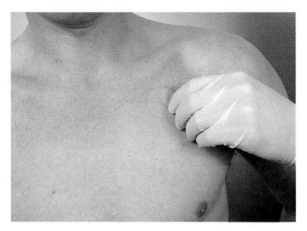

Fig. 12

Hypothermia

Victims of hypothermia have been known to be re-suscitated after prolonged exposure. It will take longer to do your assessment since you may have to feel for a pulse for up to 60 seconds. If you do not feel a pulse, begin CPR until an AED is available. Dry the victim's chest and attach the AED. If shock is indicated, first deliver three shocks. If there is still no pulse, continue CPR. Follow your local protocol as to whether additional shocks should be delivered. You should continue CPR, protect the victim from further heat loss, and remove wet garments if possible. Be sure not to defibrillate a victim in water.

Trauma and AEDs

If a person is in cardiac arrest resulting from traumatic injuries, the AED may still be used.

Defibrillation should be continued according to local protocol.

Maintenance

For defibrillators to perform optimally, they must be maintained like any other machine. The AEDs that are available today require minimal maintenance. These devices have various self-testing features. However, it is important that you are familiar with any visual or audible warning prompts your AED may have to warn of malfunction or a low battery. It is important that you read the operator's manual thoroughly and check with the manufacturer to obtain all necessary information regarding maintenance.

In most instances, if the machine detects any malfunction, you should contact the manufacturer. The device may need to be returned to the manufacturer for service.

While AEDs require minimal maintenance, it is important to remember the following:

- Follow the manufacturer's specific recommendations for periodic equipment check.
- Make sure that batteries have enough energy for one complete rescue.
- If the defibrillator is hooked up to a charger, make sure that it is charging properly.
- Make sure that defibrillator pads are in the package and properly sealed.
- Check any expiration dates on defibrillation pads and replace as needed.
- After use, make sure that all accessories are replaced and that the machine is in proper working order.

- If at any time the machine fails to work properly or warning indicators are recognized, contact the manufacturer immediately.

Establishing an Early Defibrillation Program

n early defibrillation program must consider the following variables to be successful. These variables include—

- The size, age, and location of the populations to be served.
- The number of responders being trained.
- The response times of both first responders and more advanced personnel.
- The number of AEDs available.
- Where the AEDs are placed within the community.
- The commitment to the program from the local medical director and EMS personnel.
- State and local requirements for certification in automated external defibrillation.

When these variables are taken into account, the programs established can better suit the community. For example, if an extremely large number of older adults live in the northeast section of your community, this section is where the AED should be placed. This is the area where cardiac arrests are most likely to occur. If you have several AEDs, they should be strategically placed throughout the community in areas most densely populated with your high-risk citizens so that response times can be reduced and access to defibrillation can be increased, thereby saving more lives.

Summary

Automated external defibrillators (AEDs) show great promise in saving the lives of victims of cardiac arrest. To defibrillate a victim of cardiac arrest using an AED, take the following basic steps:

1. Confirm cardiac arrest.
2. Turn on the AED.
3. Attach the AED to defibrillator pads and cables, and apply the pads to the victim's chest.
4. Let the AED analyze the heart rhythm (or push the button marked "analyze").
5. Deliver a shock if one is indicated after ensuring that no one is touching the victim and that there are no hazards present.

You must follow local protocols that establish how many shocks are delivered, the energy setting of each shock, and how CPR and other lifesaving measures are used.

AEDs are relatively easy to operate and generally require minimal training and retraining. Strategically placed in a community where the first persons to arrive on the scene are trained in their use, AEDs are a highly valuable emergency resource of great promise in saving the lives of cardiac arrest victims.

Skill Sheet: AED Basics

1. Confirm cardiac arrest (Fig. 13).

• Check pulse for 5-10 seconds.

If no pulse . . . begin CPR until AED is attached to victim.

If pulse . . . check for breathing.

2. Attach the device (Figs. 14 and 15) and turn on the AED.

• If AED has a voice recorder, give a verbal report that includes —
  • Your identity and location.
  • Assessment findings.
  • Any significant events.

• Wipe the chest dry.

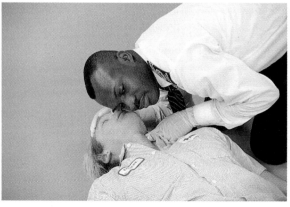

Fig. 13

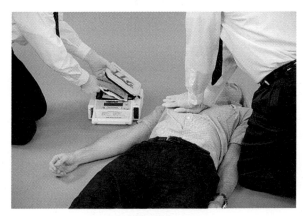

Fig. 14

- Connect cables to pads, if necessary.
- Place pads on the victim's chest.
  - Right pad goes on the right below the collar-bone.
  - Left pad goes on the left side below the nipple.

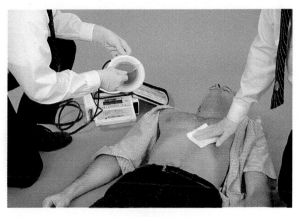

Fig. 15

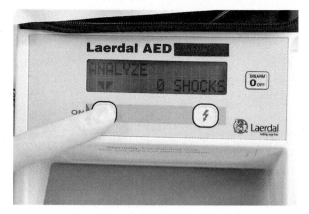

Fig. 16

3. If necessary, press analyze button (Fig. 16).

- Make sure no one is touching the victim.
- Press the button marked "analyze."

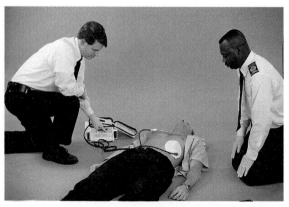

Fig. 17

If shock is indicated . . .

4. Advise rescuers and bystanders to "stand clear."

5. Deliver shock (Fig. 17).

- If the AED identifies a shockable rhythm, prepare to deliver shock.
- Instruct others to "stand clear" and make sure there are no hazards present.
- Push the shock button to defibrillate.

After delivering the shock, analyze again. Deliver another shock if indicated. Total number of shocks delivered is determined by local protocols.

If no shock is indicated . . .

- Recheck pulse, if none is found start CPR.
- After 1 minute of CPR, analyze again.

If you feel a pulse . . .

- Check breathing.

Glossary

Asystole: The absence of any electrical activity in the heart.

Atria: The two upper chambers of the heart.

Atrioventricular (AV) node: A point along the heart's electrical pathway midway between the atria and ventricles that sends electrical impulses to the ventricles.

Automated external defibrillator (AED): A semiautomatic device that recognizes a heart rhythm that requires a shock and prompts the rescuer to deliver the shock. Sometimes referred to as a semiautomatic external defibrillator (SAED).

Conduction system: Specialized cells that initiate and carry on electrical activity of the heart.

Defibrillation: An electric shock delivered to the heart to correct certain life-threatening heart rhythms.

Electrocardiogram (ECG): A graphic record produced by a device that records the electrical activity of the heart from the chest.

Electrocardiograph: A device used to record the electrical activity of the heart; a cardiac monitor.

Normal sinus rhythm: A regular heart rhythm that occurs within a normal rate, 60 to 100 beats per minute (bpm), and without unusual variations.

Purkinje fibers: A vast network of microscopic fibers that carry an electrical impulse through the ventricles.

Sinoatrial (SA) node: The normal origin of the heart's electrical impulse.

Ventricles: The two lower chambers of the heart.

Ventricular fibrillation (V-fib): A life-threatening heart rhythm; a state of totally disorganized electrical activity in the heart.

Ventricular tachycardia (V-tach): A life-threatening heart rhythm in which there is very rapid contraction of the ventricles.

Notes

Notes

Notes

Notes

Notes

Notes

Notes

Notes

MISSION OF THE AMERICAN RED CROSS

The American Red Cross, a humanitarian organization led by volunteers and guided by its Congressional Charter and the Fundamental Principles of the International Red Cross Movement, will provide relief to victims of disaster and help people prevent, prepare for, and respond to emergencies.

ABOUT THE AMERICAN RED CROSS

To support the mission of the American Red Cross, over 1.3 million paid and volunteer staff serve in some 1,600 chapters and blood centers throughout the United States and its territories and on military installations around the world. Supported by the resources of a national organization, they form the largest volunteer service and educational force in the nation. They serve families and communities through blood services, disaster relief and preparedness education services to military family members in crisis, and health and safety education.

The American Red Cross provides consistent, reliable education and training in injury and illness prevention and emergency care, providing training to nearly 16 million people each year in first aid, CPR, swimming, water safety, and HIV/AIDS education.

All of these essential services are made possible by the voluntary services, blood and tissue donations, and financial support of the American people.

FUNDAMENTAL PRINCIPLES OF THE INTERNATIONAL RED CROSS AND RED CRESCENT MOVEMENT

HUMANITY

IMPARTIALITY

NEUTRALITY

INDEPENDENCE

VOLUNTARY SERVICE

UNITY

UNIVERSALITY